DMEK *for patients*
99 of your most common questions answered

Jack S. Parker
John S. Parker
Gerrit R.J. Melles

With forward written by Ed Sweeney

Call with questions, or to schedule an appointment

Jack S. Parker MD, PhD & John S. Parker, MD
Parker Cornea
1720 University Blvd Suite 503
Birmingham, AL 35233
205-933-1077

Gerrit R.J. Melles MD, PhD
Melles Cornea Clinic and the Netherlands Institute for Innovative Ocular Surgery (NIIOS)
Laan op Zuid 88
3071 AA Rotterdam, The Netherlands
+31 10 297 4444

DMEK *for patients*: 99 of your most common questions answered

Forward - A Patient's Perspective

I came to know of the authors of this book while researching the difference between two surgery options: DSAEK and DMEK for Fuchs Dystrophy. I was diagnosed by my optician many years ago and 'lived with it' using hypertonic saline drops 5% during the progression of the disease until I decided that my sight was not allowing me to enjoy safe evening driving and even new technologies, like 4K televisions. The colors and clarity everyone touted as 'spectacular,' were just not evident to me. It was time to take action!

Deciding to go the DMEK route was an easy choice, as you will read in this book. Researching cornea specialists that specialized in the DMEK procedure led me to Parker Cornea in Birmingham, Alabama. Both Drs. Jack and John Parker work closely with Dr. Gerrit Melles, who pioneered the DMEK procedure and continues to improve it to this day at his clinic and hospital in The Netherlands. The Parkers trained under his direct supervision and Dr. Melles also visits their clinic in Birmingham, as well. I was lucky enough to meet Dr. Melles in mid-2018, in Birmingham during one of my visits following my first DMEK surgery.

Now, terms like 'transplant,' 'donor tissue,' and even 'eye surgery' make all of us nervous and apprehensive, but being informed prior to your first surgery, or even your first visit with a cornea specialist can quickly turn your apprehension into excitement.

While this book covers 99 of the most commonly asked questions, you will come away with questions that need to be addressed about your unique situation, so I cannot stress this next point enough. Ask those questions! Write a physical list of questions out before you visit any doctor you see for any condition, not just a cornea specialist.

We have all had this happen...The exam door swings open and in walks the doctor. Most people tense-up and forget many questions we only think of later that we forgot to ask, which leaves us wondering. Sometimes we turn to the internet and think the correct answer will be there. We all know, but rarely admit, that much of what we find online is either misinformation or opinion crafted to look like a fact when the doctor could have given you the correct answer face-to-face and calmed your concern right away. Don't leave the exam room with any 'what if?' unanswered and follow your all of your surgeon's post-op instructions to achieve optimum success. Vivid color and clarity will be your reward!

I believe Dr. Jack asked me to write this forword because I happen to be a 'forward' type of guy. I do not get intimidated when I encounter something I know little about. I get curious! Be curious too!

By the way, I always tell people that I experienced less discomfort during my DMEK surgeries than while having my teeth cleaned. Be excited and if you are not already, be an organ donor, as well!

Ed Sweeney is a 2018 DMEK patient who lives in Auburn, Alabama.

DMEK *for patients*: 99 of your most common questions answered

Table of Contents

FORWARD - A PATIENT'S PERSPECTIVE 3

INTRODUCTION 7

HELPFUL PICTURES 8

FUCHS DYSTROPHY 10

1. What is Fuchs dystrophy? 11
2. What are the symptoms of Fuchs dystrophy? 11
3. What causes Fuchs dystrophy? 11
4. How common is Fuchs dystrophy? 12
5. Does Fuchs dystrophy always affect both eyes? 12
6. Why is my vision worse in the morning and better as the day goes on? 12
7. Am I going to go blind? 12
8. If I have Fuchs dystrophy, does that mean my children will get it, too? 12
9. Now that I've been diagnosed, do I need to have the rest of my family checked? 12
10. It seems like my Fuchs dystrophy worsened after I had cataract surgery. Can that happen? 13
11. Does everyone with Fuchs dystrophy need a corneal transplant? 13
12. How do I know when I need a corneal transplant? 13
13. Can my Fuchs dystrophy ever come back after corneal transplantation? 13
14. What happens if I decide not to have surgery? 14
15. Are there any alternatives to surgery? What about stronger glasses? Eye drops? 14
16. Are there any online resources where I can learn more? 14

DMEK – BASIC INFORMATION 16

17. What is DMEK? 17
18. How does DMEK work? 17
19. How do you get those new cells in there? Do you have to remove my eye? 17
20. How do you get those new cells to stay put in my eye? Glue? Stitches? 17
21. What are the potential benefits of DMEK? 17
22. What is the success rate of the surgery? 18
23. How is DMEK different from other kinds of corneal transplantation (like DSAEK) 18
24. I've heard that not all corneal specialists do DMEK. Why not? 18
25. What qualifications should my corneal surgeon have? 18
26. Why not just replace the whole cornea, instead? 18
27. Who invented DMEK, and when? 19
28. Is everyone with Fuchs dystrophy a candidate for DMEK? 19
29. What if I've already had some kind of corneal surgery before. Am I still a candidate? ... 19
30. Am I too old to have surgery? 19

DMEK – BEFORE SURGERY 21

31. When I come for my initial consultation, it seems like you're doing a lot of tests. Why? 22
32. If both my eyes need a DMEK, can they both be done on the same day? 23
33. Do I need to stop my blood thinners before surgery? 23
34. What do I need to make sure the doctor knows about me before my surgery? 23
35. Is my insurance going to cover the operation? If so, what's my copay going to be? .. 24
36. How long should I be off work after surgery? 24
37. Tell me what happens to me on the day of my surgery – what's the day like? 24

DMEK *for patients*: 99 of your most common questions answered

DMEK – DURING SURGERY 26
- 38. How do you do the surgery? 27
- 39. How long does the surgery take? 27
- 40. Will I be asleep during the surgery? 27
- 41. Does the surgery hurt? 27
- 42. What if I have a cataract, too? Can that be removed at the same time? 28
- 43. Do I have to stay overnight in the hospital? 28
- 44. What are the biggest risks of the surgery? 28
- 45. I'd like to watch my surgery. Do you videotape the operation and, if so, can I get a copy? 28

DMEK – AFTER SURGERY 30
- 46. Immediately after the surgery, what should I be feeling? 31
- 47. … what should I be seeing? 31
- 48. … what should I be doing? 31
- 49. What's the single most important thing for me to do after the surgery? 31
- 50. Do I really have to lie on my back for two days after the surgery? Can I lie in a recliner, instead? 32
- 51. I'm driving from far away; I'm worried about not being able to lie down during my ride home. 32
- 52. Overall, what's the recovery period? 32
- 53. What kind of vision can I expect to get back after the operation? 32
- 54. Will I need new glasses after surgery? If so, how soon can I get them? 33
- 55. Can I wear contact lenses after DMEK? If so, when? 33
- 56. After surgery, will my eye look any different? Are people going to know that I've had surgery? 33
- 57. After surgery, do I need to come back to the office for checkups? If so, how often? 33
- 58. Can I just see my regular eye doctor after the surgery, or do I have to come back and see you? 34
- 59. What restrictions do I have after surgery? What can't I do? 34
- 60. How long after the surgery until I can fly? 34
- 61. … until I can exercise? 34
- 62. … until I can swim? 34
- 63. Do I have to wear an eye patch after surgery? If so, for how long? 34
- 64. Do I need to use eye drops after surgery? If so, what kind and for how long? 35
- 65. How much are these drops going to cost me? 35
- 66. What happens if I stop using my drops? 35
- 67. Is it okay for me to try stopping my drops? 35
- 68. Can these drops ever cause any problems? 35
- 69. When I come back for my post-operative visits, what are you checking for? 36
- 70. Do I really need all these tests? 37
- 71. I've heard about "graft detachments." What are those? How common are they? 37
- 72. How can I tell if my graft is detached? 37
- 73. How does my doctor tell if my graft is detached? 37
- 74. What can I do after surgery to prevent my graft from detaching? 37
- 75. What happens if I develop a graft detachment? Do I have to go back to surgery? 37
- 76. If I develop a graft detachment in my first eye, does that mean my other eye will, too? 38
- 77. I've heard that some doctors use special gasses with DMEK surgery to help the graft attach. Why? 38
- 78. What happens if my graft is discovered to be "upside-down" after surgery? 38
- 79. If we have to go back to surgery to fix a problem, will my insurance pay for that? 38
- 80. Can my corneal transplant ever "reject"? If so, then what happens? Can it be treated? 38
- 81. How can I tell if I am having a graft rejection? 39
- 82. How does my doctor tell if I am having a graft rejection? 39
- 83. My surgery was years ago…does that mean I'm safe from rejection? 39
- 84. Is there anything I can do to prevent my graft from rejecting? 39
- 85. If the doctor can't stop the rejection and my transplant fails, then what happens? 39
- 86. How long does a corneal transplant last? Forever, or will it need to be repeated? 40

87. WHERE DO YOU GET THE DONOR CORNEAL TISSUE FROM? 40
88. CAN YOU TELL ME ABOUT THE DONOR THAT MY CORNEAL TRANSPLANT IS COMING FROM? 40
89. CAN I PICK MY OWN DONOR TISSUE? 40
90. CAN I STILL BE AN ORGAN DONOR IF HAVE THIS SURGERY? 40
91. SINCE THE SURGERY, I'VE NOTICED THAT MY EYE FEELS SCRATCHY SOMETIMES. IS THAT NORMAL? 40
92. SINCE THE SURGERY, I'VE NOTICED THAT I CAN SEE A BLACK DOT ON MY EYE. WHAT IS THAT? 41
93. MY SURGERY WAS YEARS AGO, AND EVERYTHING HAS BEEN FINE, BUT LATELY MY EYE HAS BEEN RED AND HURTING. WHAT SHOULD I DO? 41
94. HOW SOON AFTER THE FIRST EYE CAN THE SECOND EYE BE OPERATED ON? 41
95. AFTER I HAVE THIS SURGERY, DOES THIS MEAN I NEED TO SEE A CORNEAL SPECIALIST FOREVER? 41
96. I'VE HEARD THAT FUCHS DYSTROPHY CAN BE TREATED IN SOME PATIENTS BY JUST SCRAPING THE BACK OF THE CORNEA, AND NOT DOING A TRANSPLANT AT ALL. IS THAT TRUE, AND IF SO, AM I CANDIDATE FOR THIS PROCEDURE? 41
97. IS THERE ANYTHING NEW COMING UP THAT WOULD BE BETTER THAN DMEK? SHOULD I WAIT? 42
98. I'D LIKE TO DONATE TO THE RESEARCH EFFORTS OF DR. MELLES. WHERE CAN I DO THAT? 42
99. ARE THERE ANY OTHER BOOKS ON THE SUBJECT OF DMEK THAT I MIGHT FIND INTERESTING OR USEFUL? 42

Introduction

DMEK is the newest, most advanced form of corneal transplantation in the world. It offers the best visual results, the most rapid recovery, and the fewest risks. The operation is quick, painless, and minimally invasive – no stitches, no bleeding, and usually not even an eye patch

But, as wonderful as this procedure can be, achieving a good result always requires a cooperative effort between doctor and patient. That's why we've written this book – to take our time, and carefully explain all the important details of your surgery, including what you can expect before, during, and after your operation in Birmingham, AL.

Here, we've tried to cover it all. Of course, everybody's different, and no two patient experiences are exactly the same. But, in these pages, we've tried hard to put all the facts on the table and to write the book that we'd want to read, if it were us having the surgery.

Jack Parker, John Parker, & Gerrit Melles

Helpful pictures

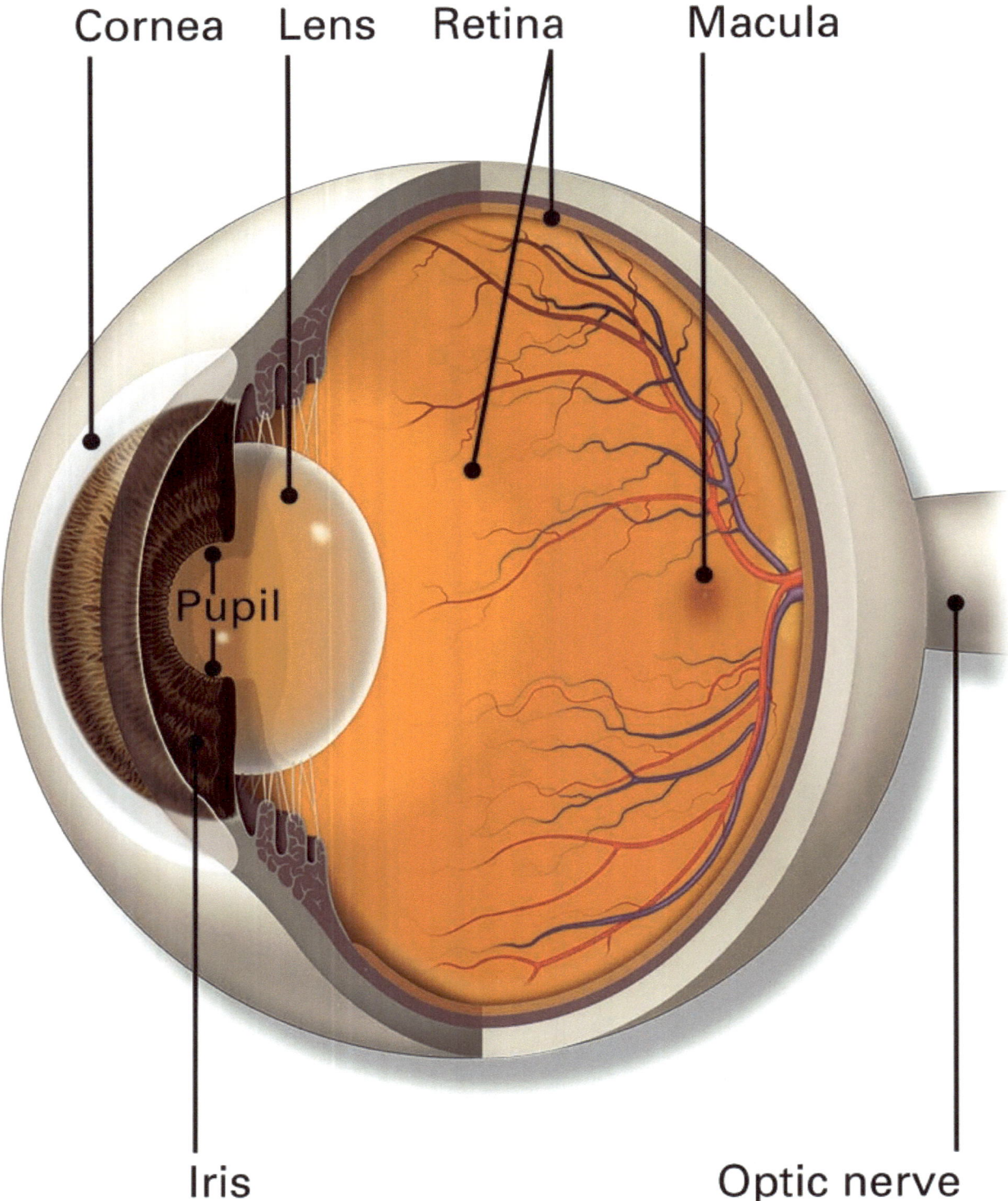

Image © American Academy of Ophthalmology

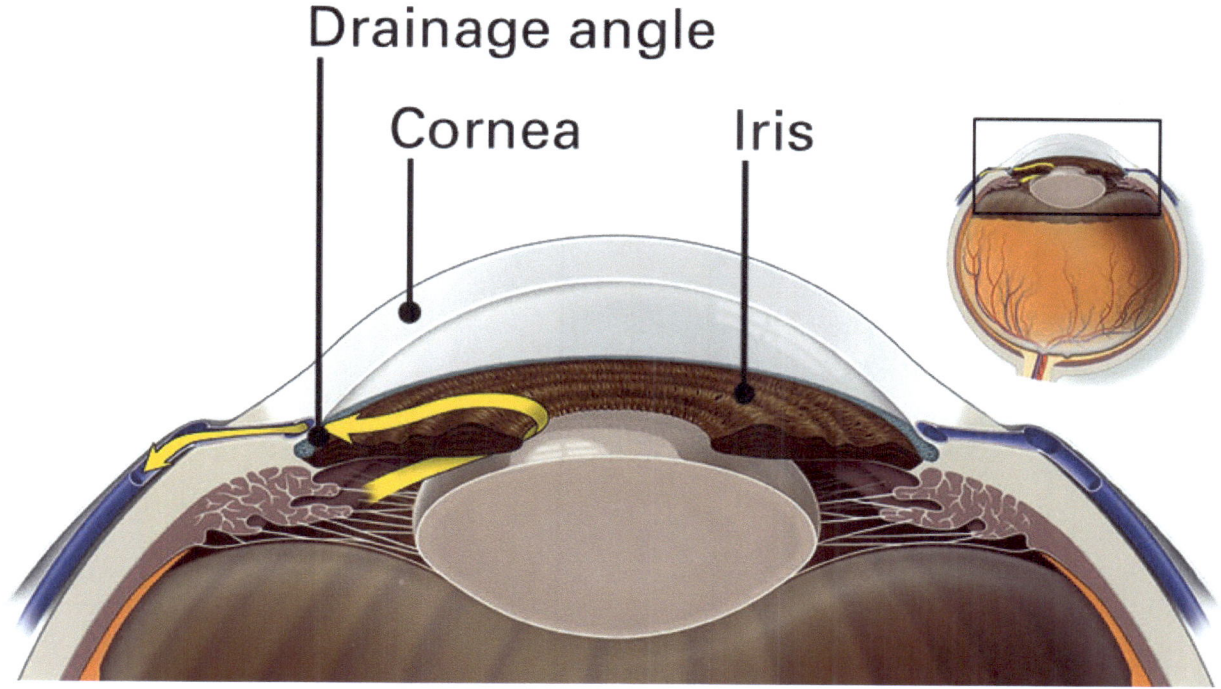

Image © American Academy of Ophthalmology

Fuchs Dystrophy

1. What is Fuchs dystrophy?

Fuchs dystrophy is a common disease of the back of the cornea. Normally, thousands and thousands of little pump cells live back there. Their job is to keep the cornea thin and clear.

But, in Fuchs dystrophy, tiny bumps (called guttae) start to appear. They grow around, underneath, and in between the cornea's pump cells. It's like a garden slowly being taken over by weeds.

As the bumps multiply, the cornea's pump cells die, the cornea becomes hazy, and the whole thing starts to swell. Then your vision gets cloudy, and your eye can even start to hurt.

In your garden, you can sometimes get rid of weeds just by pulling them out. But in Fuchs dystrophy, there are so many of these little bumps, we often end up having to replace the whole lawn to get rid of them. We call that a corneal transplant.

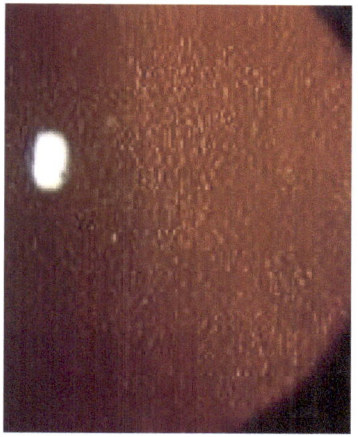 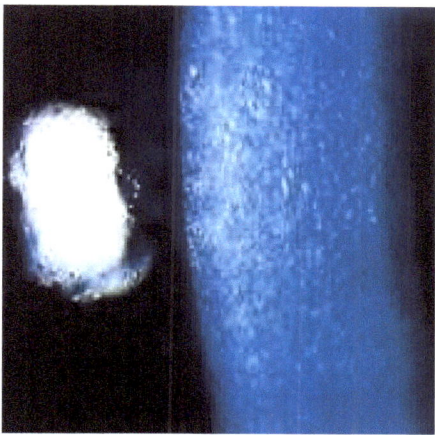 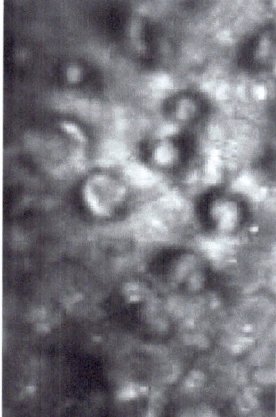

2. What are the symptoms of Fuchs dystrophy?

You may notice that your vision is not as sharp as it used to be. Things may appear dim or out of focus, and you may have trouble seeing to do things that you were formerly able to accomplish easily. Some patients complain about difficulty reading, sewing, or driving at night. Colors may appear "washed out." Glare and halos around lights may become noticeable. In the morning, things may be especially bad.

3. What causes Fuchs dystrophy?

No one knows. It's probably partially genetic, which means that it can run in some families, but not always.

4. How common is Fuchs dystrophy?

   Estimates vary, but several studies have reported that about 4% of people 50 years or older may show signs of the disease.

5. Does Fuchs dystrophy always affect both eyes?

   Yes, but the disease is often worse in one eye.

6. Why is my vision worse in the morning and better as the day goes on?

   With Fuchs dystrophy, the cornea's pump cells have trouble keeping fluid out, so the cornea tends to swell. During the daytime, when you have your eyes open, fluid evaporates into the air, so your pump cells have help getting rid of water. But at night when you close your eyes and go to bed, fluid can't evaporate through your eyelids. So, while you're sleeping, your corneas swell up. In the morning when you open your eyes, things will probably look extra blurry. As the day goes on and you have your eyes open, evaporation helps you get rid of some of that fluid again, and your vision improves a bit.

7. Am I going to go blind?

   Fortunately, that's extremely unlikely. Fuchs Dystrophy is curable.

8. If I have Fuchs dystrophy, does that mean my children will get it, too?

   Not necessarily. There are lots of families in which only one person, or only a few people, are affected.

   Fortunately, even if your children do inherit the disease from you, usually Fuchs dystrophy doesn't cause any problems until the patient is middle-aged or older.

9. Now that I've been diagnosed, do I need to have the rest of my family checked?

   If they're adults, it probably wouldn't hurt. It can be important for them know if they have Fuchs dystrophy before undergoing any other type of eye surgery (cataract removal, for example) which can sometimes make Fuchs dystrophy worse.

10. It seems like my Fuchs dystrophy worsened after I had cataract surgery. Can that happen?

    Unfortunately, yes. Sometimes, even after perfectly performed cataract surgery, your cornea can swell, and your vision can become cloudy, especially if you have Fuchs dystrophy.

11. Does everyone with Fuchs dystrophy need a corneal transplant?

    No. Some people are lucky enough to have a mild form of the disease that doesn't require any treatment.

12. How do I know when I need a corneal transplant?

    You might need a corneal transplant if:

    1) Your vision is not good enough to do the things you want or need to do.

    – or –

    2) Your cornea is starting to swell.

    The first reason is self-explanatory. If you're having trouble seeing, things are not going to get any better on their own – they're only going to get worse.

    The second reason takes a little bit more explaining. As your Fuchs dystrophy worsens, your cornea may start to swell. At this point, even if your vision is ok, this can still be a problem. Having a soggy, swollen cornea is not good for your eye – it's like having standing water in the basement of your house. You can't leave it there, or you're going to end up with permanent problems. So, if your cornea starts to swell, you might need a corneal transplant, even if your vision is not that bad.

    Corneal swelling is not usually something you can detect on your own – you'll probably need to see a corneal specialist to know for sure whether you've got it.

13. Can my Fuchs dystrophy ever come back after corneal transplantation?

    No. Once it's gone, it's gone for good.

14. What happens if I decide not to have surgery?

Your vision will probably continue to decline. If your cornea starts to swell, and you still don't receive a transplant, you may get blisters on your cornea, and then your cornea may start to scar. These changes are usually slow, but they're bad, and they're not always reversible.

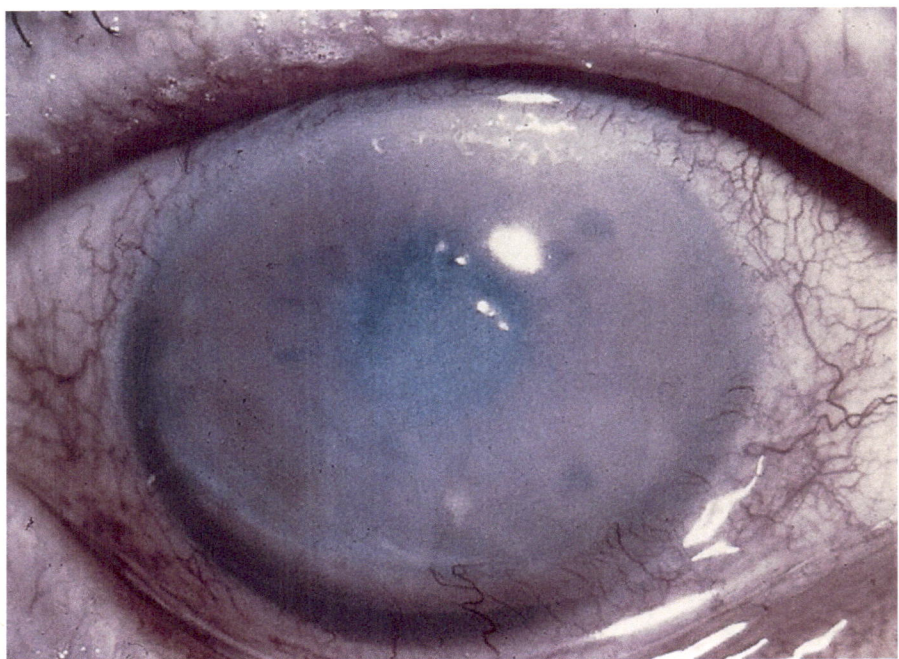

Image © American Academy of Ophthalmology

15. Are there any alternatives to surgery? What about stronger glasses? Eye drops?

Unfortunately, none of these other things work. The only effective treatment is surgery.

There is an over-the-counter eyedrop called Muro 128 (hypertonic saline), and it's basically a salt water solution that can dry your corneas out. In some people, this can lessen the symptoms of Fuchs dystrophy, but it does not stop the disease from progressing.

16. Are there any online resources where I can learn more?

The best website that we know of is "Fuchs Friends" which is an online forum run by patients with Fuchs dystrophy, many of whom have already had surgery and can give you valuable information about what to expect.

DMEK – basic information

17. What is DMEK?

DMEK stands for "Descemet membrane endothelial keratoplasty."

DMEK is a kind of corneal transplant surgery in which only the back layer of the cornea is replaced.

18. How does DMEK work?

The cells that live on the back of your cornea are very important – they're little pumps, and they work hard to keep your cornea thin and clear. If something happens to those pump cells, then your cornea can become swollen and cloudy.

DMEK is pump-cell replacement surgery. The operation involves a "graft" which is a set of pump cells taken from a healthy donor eye that are "transplanted" into your eye. These new cells now live inside your eye and work for you, to keep your cornea thin and clear, and to help you see.

You might hear your doctor talking about your "new cells" or your "graft" or your "transplant." These are all the same thing.

19. How do you get those new cells in there? Do you have to remove my eye?

Fortunately, we do not have to remove your eye. Instead, all we do is inject your new cells through a very tiny incision in your cornea, only three millimeters long. That's smaller than the eye of a needle!

20. How do you get those new cells to stay put in my eye? Glue? Stitches?

At the end of your surgery, we leave an air-bubble inside of your eye. That bubble holds your new cells against the back of your cornea until they can stick there on their own. The bubble dissolves by itself after just a few days. We don't normally use any glue or stitches.

21. What are the potential benefits of DMEK?

Most people see significantly better after DMEK. That means sharper vision, enhanced contrast, and brighter colors. This may help you watch TV, drive, play golf, read, and do many other things.

22. What is the success rate of the surgery?

For most people, the chances that we can eliminate your Fuchs dystrophy and implant a healthy set of new pump cells is greater than 95%.

23. How is DMEK different from other kinds of corneal transplantation (like DSAEK)

DMEK is an even swap – we remove the pump cells from your eye that aren't working, and we replace them with a new set of healthy cells that do work.

There's a surgery that's similar to DMEK that you may hear about – it's called DSAEK, and it's another kind of corneal transplant.

The difference is that DSAEK uses a much thicker graft than DMEK. That extra thickness is not a good thing – it makes the graft more of a target for your immune system, so you may be more likely to have problems with rejection after the surgery. The extra thickness of the graft also somewhat blocks the transmission of light through the cornea, so your vision after DSAEK probably won't be as good as your vision after DMEK.

24. I've heard that not all corneal specialists do DMEK. Why not?

DMEK is a newer surgery, and not all corneal specialists have learned how to do it yet. It also can be a more challenging operation to perform, and not all surgeons are comfortable learning a more difficult technique.

25. What qualifications should my corneal surgeon have?

You definitely want them to know how to do DMEK, and ideally to have a lot of practice doing it. A few studies suggest that it takes about 25 practice cases for a surgeon to get the hang of things.

26. Why not just replace the whole cornea, instead?

Whole-corneal replacement is not a good surgery. It's a huge, dangerous operation that permanently weakens the eye, and requires us to put a bunch of stitches in your cornea that must remain in-place for years. After a whole-corneal transplant, the eye never looks normal and never sees normally.

DMEK, on the other hand, requires no stitches. The surgery is much safer, and the eye usually looks normal and sees normally very quickly after the surgery.

27. Who invented DMEK, and when?

DMEK was invented in 1998 by a young Dutch Ophthalmologist named Gerrit Melles. Dr. Melles is still practicing and doing surgery in his clinic in Rotterdam, The Netherlands at the Melles Cornea Clinic. He is also the director of the Netherlands Institute for Innovative Ocular Surgery (NIIOS), which is among the foremost corneal research organizations in the world. Their website is: www.niios.com

28. Is everyone with Fuchs dystrophy a candidate for DMEK?

The vast majority of people with Fuchs dystrophy are good DMEK candidates. Exceptions include people with extreme corneal clouding, or people with severe iris or lens abnormalities.

29. What if I've already had some kind of corneal surgery before. Am I still a candidate?

Usually, the answer is still yes.

30. Am I too old to have surgery?

We've operated on people 100+ years old. You are never too old to see.

DMEK – before surgery

31. When I come for my initial consultation, it seems like you're doing a lot of tests. Why?

In addition to a complete eye exam, there are a few specialized tests you may receive when you come to the office for a surgical consultation. These include:

1) <u>Specular microscopy</u>: this is where we take pictures of the back of your cornea. We use these pictures to check the health of your pump cells and look for diseases like Fuchs dystrophy.

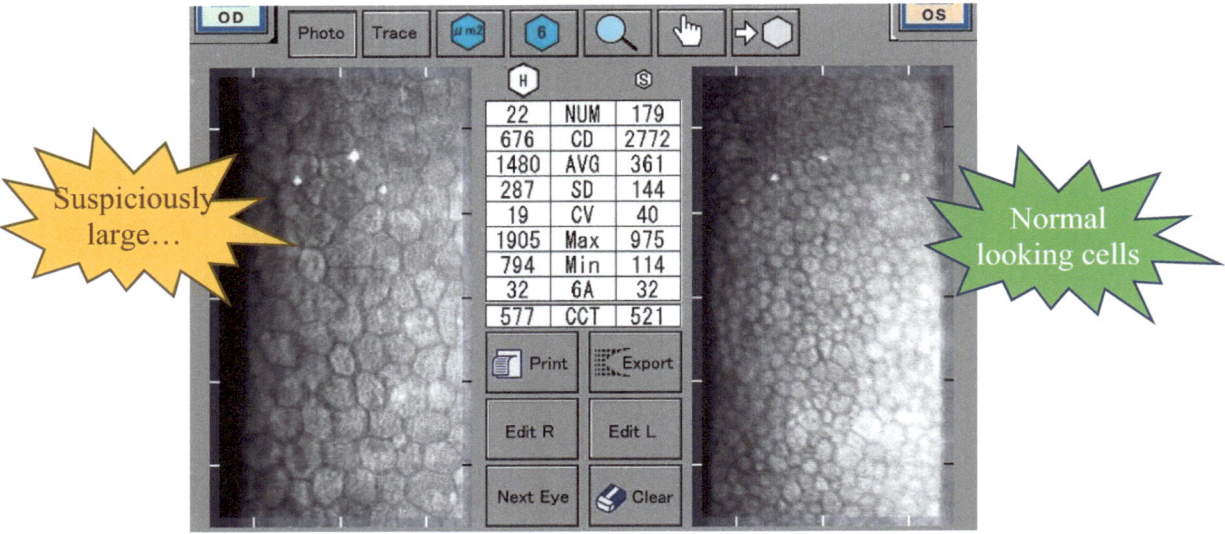

2) <u>Pentacam imaging</u>: this is where we measure the thickness and shape of your cornea, which helps us with our surgical planning.

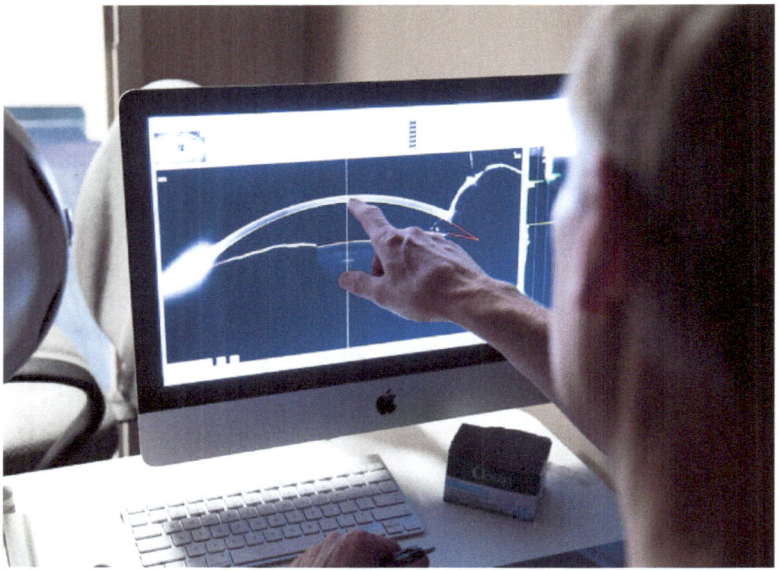

32. If both my eyes need a DMEK, can they both be done on the same day?

No, we only operate on one eye at a time. Generally, we start with your worse-seeing eye. If that operation goes well and your vision improves, we can schedule surgery for your second eye. Generally, we wait at least two weeks after the first eye before operating on the second eye.

33. Do I need to stop my blood thinners before surgery?

Yes, if:

1) You are taking a prescription blood thinner like aspirin, Coumadin, Plavix, or Eliquis

– and –

2) You receive permission from your cardiologist, internal medicine, or primary care doctor to temporarily discontinue the medicine.

Stopping your blood thinners before the surgery can reduce your chances of bleeding during the operation, but you should not discontinue your medications without prior permission from your medical doctor. If you are unable to discontinue your blood thinners, your surgery can almost always be done safely, regardless.

Ideally, aspirin, Coumadin, and Plavix should be stopped 5 days before surgery; Eliquis should be stopped 2 days before surgery. All medications can be resumed the day after your operation.

34. What do I need to make sure the doctor knows about me before my surgery?

The three most important things for your doctor to know about you before your surgery are:

1) Whether you have any history of viral infection in *either eye*, especially Herpes virus infections (simplex, zoster, or cytomegalovirus). This is very important because you may need to be treated before your surgery to prevent the virus from recurring after your operation.
2) Whether you are currently taking any blood thinners.
3) Whether you are unable to lie flat on your back for at least an hour at a time.

35. Is my insurance going to cover the operation? If so, what's my copay going to be?

Yes, your insurance will pay for the surgery. Your copay depends on the insurance plan that you have.

36. How long should I be off work after surgery?

That depends on what you do for a living and how quickly you heal after the operation. Everyone's different but you can expect to be out of work for one week.

37. Tell me what happens to me on the day of my surgery – what's the day like?

You'll show up to the hospital on the morning of your surgery. Check in at admissions, and you'll head to the pre-operative area, along with your family or friends or anyone else who came with you that day.

In pre-op, you'll change into your hospital gown, an IV will be started in your arm, and you'll start receiving some eye drops in the eye that's scheduled for surgery.

Then your doctors will come by. We'll chat with you about the operation, give you a wrist-band, and put a mark over the eye scheduled for surgery.

When your operating room is ready, you'll get one last chance to stop by the restroom, and then we'll take you back. At this point, your friends/ family will head to the waiting room.

Then we do your surgery.

After surgery, we wheel you out of the operating room to the recovery area. You'll stay in the recovery area for about 60-90 minutes, lying flat on your back, to help your graft attach. When that time is up, we'll rejoin your friends/ family, and head to a little "treatment room" to check the position of your graft using a microscope. At that point, if everything looks good, we'll give you an eye shield, and you're on your way home.

DMEK – during surgery

38. How do you do the surgery?

Very carefully!

There are a lot of videos on YouTube that you can watch. Just search for "DMEK."

Basically, what we do is: numb the area around the eye, then make a small incision in your cornea. Very carefully, we peel the sick cells away from the back of your cornea and remove them. Then, we take your new cells and bring them into your eye using a glass tube. We transfer those cells onto the back of your cornea using an air bubble. At the end of the surgery, we leave the air bubble inside your eye to help hold your new cells in place.

39. How long does the surgery take?

Between 15 and 30 minutes, on average.

40. Will I be asleep during the surgery?

No. But you will get some medicine to help you relax and stay comfortable

41. Does the surgery hurt?

No. Before we do anything, we give you some numbing medicine around the eye. During the actual operation, you might feel a little pressure and some cool water, but you shouldn't feel any pain.

42. What if I have a cataract, too? Can that be removed at the same time?

Yes, we can remove your cataract at the same time as your DMEK. That's very common and we do it all the time.

Sometimes, however, it's better to leave the cataract alone during your DMEK, and go back after it later, in a second surgery. The biggest reason that we would do that is if you have a lot of astigmatism, and you want an "astigmatism correcting" specialty lens placed in your eye when the cataract is removed.

"Astigmatism correcting" lenses require very accurate measurements to be made of your eye. These measurements depend on the health of your cornea, and if your cornea is not healthy (like, if you have Fuchs dystrophy) then these measurements can be wrong. That means we could accidentally put the wrong lens in your eye during the cataract surgery. You don't want that, and neither do we.

So, if you want an astigmatism correcting lens, it's sometimes better to get the cornea healthy first, then take good measurements, then do the cataract surgery.

This can be a complicated decision and you should talk with your doctor about what's best for your eye.

43. Do I have to stay overnight in the hospital?

Not usually; most of the time you can leave the hospital within two hours of the end of your surgery.

44. What are the biggest risks of the surgery?

Bleeding and infection are the two main ones, both of which are uncommon but potentially very serious. Rarely, we may be unable to implant the donor cells during the operation; after the operation, your body's immune system may reject the transplant. Your eye pressure might increase after the surgery. To fix these problems, more surgery may be necessary.

45. I'd like to watch my surgery. Do you videotape the operation and, if so, can I get a copy?

Many surgeons record their operations, and they might be glad to share pictures or videos of your case with you, if you ask.

DMEK – after surgery

46. Immediately after the surgery, what should I be feeling?

The eye will probably feel watery and scratchy and stingy, and you may prefer to keep it closed. It shouldn't be really aching you, like a toothache or an ice cream headache. When you leave the hospital, if you'll take a little nap, that will probably help.

47. ... what should I be seeing?

Right after your surgery, you won't be able to see hardly anything out of your operated eye. *That's normal.* And, it's because of three things:

1) The numbing medicine we give you temporarily prevents the eye from seeing.

2) Your new cells are kept in the refrigerator in a storage solution before your surgery, and it takes a few days for them to "wake up" and start working after your operation.

3) We leave a large air-bubble in your eye to hold your new cells in place against the back of your cornea. That bubble takes a few days to dissolve. Until then, you'll be looking through it, which can make things extra blurry.

48. ... what should I be doing?

Wear your eye shield so you don't accidentally rub your eye, especially while you're sleeping. As much as possible, try to remain flat on your back facing the ceiling for the first 48 hours after the operation to help your new cells attach securely to the back of your cornea.

49. What's the single most important thing for me to do after the surgery?

On the day of your surgery, the number one most important thing to remember is this: When you go home, it's normal for your eye to be itchy or scratchy or watery, but it shouldn't hurt you really bad, like a toothache or an ice cream headache. If it does, that could mean that the pressure in your eye is too high, and you need to call your doctor immediately! The first 24 hours are the most important, and if you have this symptom, you need to call right away, even if it's 3am, so it can get fixed.

50. Do I really have to lie on my back for two days after the surgery? Can I lie in a recliner, instead?

A recliner is fine. And, you can take breaks to eat, go to the bathroom, shower, and stretch. Don't make yourself miserable. But as much as you are comfortably able, try to lie back to help your new cells settle into their new home.

51. I'm driving from far away; I'm worried about not being able to lie down during my ride home.

We hear that all the time, and it's not a problem. For patients traveling from more than an hour away, we recommend you plan on spending the night after surgery in a local hotel. For patients traveling less than one hour, it's ok to sit up in the car with your seatbelt on.

52. Overall, what's the recovery period?

For the first few days after the surgery, your vision will be very blurry in the operated eye. During this time, it's also normal for the eye to feel a little watery and scratchy, and like you've got something in it.

For the first 48 hours, you'll be asked to lay flat on your back looking at the ceiling as much as you are comfortably able, to help your new cells stick to the back of your cornea.

A few days after the surgery, you should notice that the vision in your operated eye is starting to clear up, and your eye is starting to feel more comfortable.

About a week after the surgery, you'll probably feel and see well enough to return to work and to most of your hobbies and activities, although it may take several months for your vision to reach its final level.

53. What kind of vision can I expect to get back after the operation?

When a cornea swells, a gradual loss of transparency develops. This loss of transparency, depending on how severe it is and how long it has been present, can limit your vision even after DMEK. Even so, assuming that there are no other problems with your eye, you have at least a 50% chance of getting 20/20 vision (or better) after your operation.

Everybody's different, but around 1-2 weeks after the surgery, most people are seeing better than they were before the operation.

54. Will I need new glasses after surgery? If so, how soon can I get them?

Many people do benefit from an updated glasses prescription after DMEK. If you need a new pair, those are usually given around 3 months after your surgery by your regular eye doctor.

55. Can I wear contact lenses after DMEK? If so, when?

Many people benefit from an updated contact lens prescription, which you can get (on average) 3 months after your DMEK from your regular eye doctor.

56. After surgery, will my eye look any different? Are people going to know that I've had surgery?

You won't look any different, and no one will know unless you tell them.

57. After surgery, do I need to come back to the office for checkups? If so, how often?

In the first couple weeks after surgery, you'll probably see your surgeon a few times to make sure that your new cells are where they're supposed to be. After that, you'll need to come back much less often – once a year, or even less.

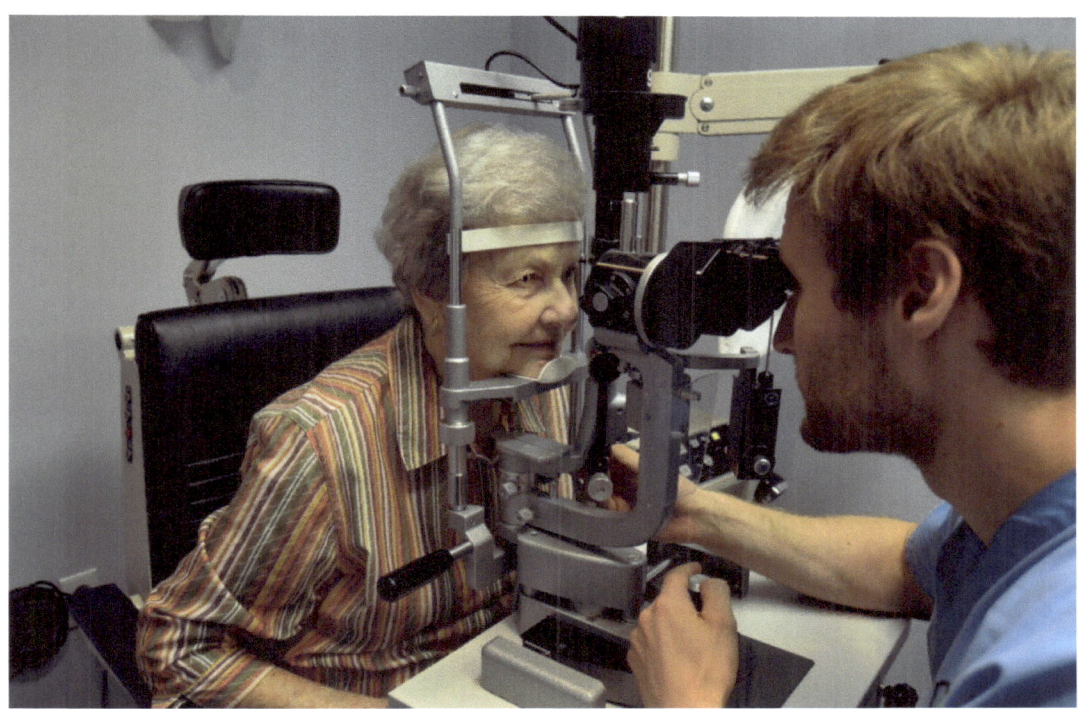

58. Can I just see my regular eye doctor after the surgery, or do I have to come back and see you?

Generally, your surgeon will want to see you a few times after the surgery, so we can make sure your new cells look ok. After that, you're free to return to your regular eye doctor for your checkups.

59. What restrictions do I have after surgery? What can't I do?

We want you to lie flat on your back as much as possible for the first 48 hours after surgery. We also like you to sleep with an eye shield for the first few days after the operation, so you don't accidentally rub your eye in your sleep. In general, it's good to avoid heavy lifting (anything more than 20 pounds) for one week.

60. How long after the surgery until I can fly?

Probably, you could get on a plane the very next day, if you really wanted to. But, make sure you're around for your post-operative visits, especially that first week.

61. ... until I can exercise?

Walking for exercise is okay 3 days after the surgery; running is okay at 2 weeks, and weight lifting at 4 weeks.

62. ... until I can swim?

One month

63. Do I have to wear an eye patch after surgery? If so, for how long?

You may go home with a patch the day of your surgery; otherwise, an eye patch is usually not necessary. Although, your doctor may ask you to sleep with an eye shield at night for the first week after your operation.

64. Do I need to use eye drops after surgery? If so, what kind and for how long?

Yes. After your surgery, you'll probably be using at least two drops – an antibiotic and a steroid. The antibiotic is to prevent infection, and the steroid is to keep your body's immune system from rejecting your new cells. The antibiotic can often be stopped one week after your surgery. You'll may need to keep using your anti-rejection steroid eye drops forever to prevent your new transplant from rejecting.

65. How much are these drops going to cost me?

It depends on your what kind of insurance you have, and what kind of drops your doctor decides to use. Generic medications can usually be found at very reasonable cash prices near you using an app like GoodRx.

66. What happens if I stop using my drops?

Sometimes nothing, especially if it's been a long time (years) since your surgery. But lots of bad things could happen – for example, your body can start rejecting your transplant, and then your new cells could die.

67. Is it okay for me to try stopping my drops?

This is not an experiment that we typically recommend. If you stop your anti-rejection drops, your body can start attacking your transplanted cells. Even if your eye feels fine and your vision is great, your new cells can suffer permanent damage before you even realize there is a problem.

If your new cells die, then you're going to need more surgery to replace them. At that point, even if you start your drops again, the damage is already done.

68. Can these drops ever cause any problems?

Unfortunately, yes. Steroid eye drops can sometimes increase your eye pressure. If untreated, high eye pressure can cause glaucoma.

If your eye pressure starts to increase while using steroid drops, your doctor may need to reduce your dose, or change which kind of drop you are taking. Occasionally, it may be necessary to use pressure-lowering drops for some time after DMEK.

69. When I come back for my post-operative visits, what are you checking for?

In the first couple weeks after your surgery, the key thing that we're checking is that your new cells are in the right place. The problem is, those cells are too small for us to see with our eyes, even with our best microscopes. The only way for us to tell whether they're in the right place is using some very specialized imaging equipment. Your insurance may, or may not, pay for us to use this equipment. If not, the cost to you is about $35 per visit.

After those first couple weeks, the biggest things that we continue to check for are:

1) That your body isn't rejecting your new cells

– and –

2) That your anti-rejection eye drops aren't causing any problems

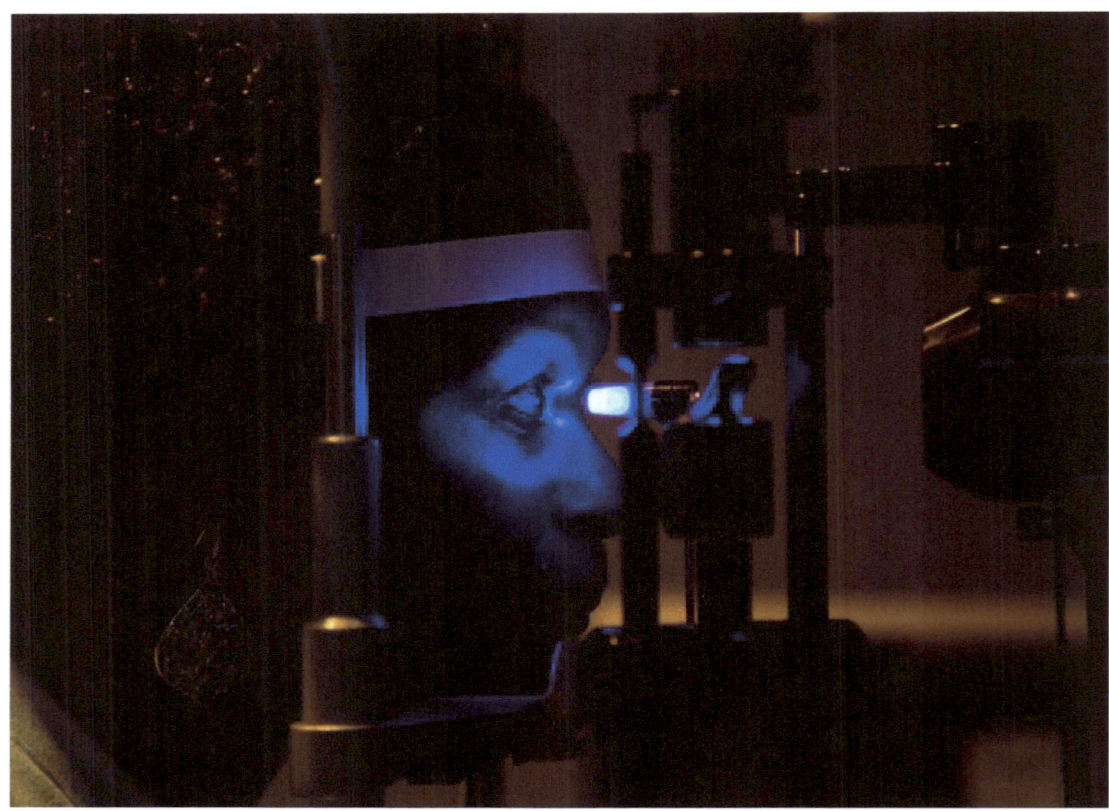

70. Do I really need all these tests?

Definitely. Hopefully, corneal transplantation is something you'll only have to go through once in your life, and it's important that we do everything to make sure you have the best results and get the best vision possible.

71. I've heard about "graft detachments." What are those? How common are they?

A graft detachment is when the new cells that we put in your eye don't stick to the back of your cornea. That happens about 10% of the time. If you're in that unlucky 10%, it's usually not a big deal, and we can get the cells back where they belong just by putting a little bit more air in the eye. Almost always, we can do that in the clinic, without needing to go back to surgery.

72. How can I tell if my graft is detached?

As the patient, you might not be able to. One possible sign is if your vision does not begin to clear up in the first couple weeks after your surgery.

73. How does my doctor tell if my graft is detached?

Occasionally, we can tell if the graft is detached by looking at your cornea with a high-powered microscope. Usually, however, we need to use specialized imaging equipment that shows the back of your cornea in super-high detail. We call that imaging technology "anterior-segment OCT."

74. What can I do after surgery to prevent my graft from detaching?

The most important thing you can do is to lie as flat on your back as possible for 48 hours after the operation, so the air bubble inside your eye can stick those cells to the back of your cornea.

75. What happens if I develop a graft detachment? Do I have to go back to surgery?

Usually, we can fix detachments just by giving you a larger air bubble. That can almost always be done in the clinic, without going back to surgery.

76. If I develop a graft detachment in my first eye, does that mean my other eye will, too?

Not necessarily, and – in fact – not usually.

77. I've heard that some doctors use special gasses with DMEK surgery to help the graft attach. Why?

It's true, there are gasses other than air (like, for example, a special sulfur and fluoride mixture) that may be more effective than air alone at sticking the pump cells to the back of your cornea. Research using these other gasses is still ongoing, and they may carry some additional risks that air does not. You might discuss this detail with your doctor if you want to know the latest on the subject.

78. What happens if my graft is discovered to be "upside-down" after surgery?

This is rare but can happen. After surgery, if we notice that your graft is flipped completely upside down, then we have to go back to surgery to fix it.

79. If we have to go back to surgery to fix a problem, will my insurance pay for that?

Every insurance plan is different. Very often though, there is an additional copay that your insurance will require you to pay, which will be similar to your copay for the original operation.

80. Can my corneal transplant ever "reject"? If so, then what happens? Can it be treated?

Yes. Your body's immune system can sometimes attack your new cells, mistaking them for an infection. We call that a "rejection." Usually, we can prevent and even reverse a graft rejection by giving you additional steroid eye drops.

81. How can I tell if I am having a graft rejection?

After surgery, if your eye becomes red, light sensitive, irritated, or if your vision starts to decline, you may be having a graft rejection, especially if you have not been taking any anti-rejection eye drops. But sometimes, a graft rejection can occur without you having any symptoms at all, which is why it is important for you to have regular checkups with your eye doctors, so they can look and make sure you don't get into this kind of trouble.

82. How does my doctor tell if I am having a graft rejection?

One way is by measuring the thickness of your cornea. After your transplant, if your cornea starts to show signs of thickening, that can be one clue that a graft rejection is starting.

We can also look directly at your transplanted cells with some very detailed pictures. These pictures can show us whether your new cells are healthy, or whether your body's immune system is attacking them.

83. My surgery was years ago...does that mean I'm safe from rejection?

No! In fact, the most common time for a graft to reject is 1-2 years after your surgery. That means you always need to pay attention and be on the lookout for trouble.

84. Is there anything I can do to prevent my graft from rejecting?

Use your steroid eye drops as directed, and if you have problems after your transplant, don't sit around and wait for them to get worse. Call or come in immediately so your doctor can examine you.

85. If the doctor can't stop the rejection and my transplant fails, then what happens?

If we can't stop your body from rejecting your new cells, eventually they might die. If so, then they'll need to be replaced with some more cells. That means another corneal transplant.

86. How long does a corneal transplant last? Forever, or will it need to be repeated?

How long a corneal transplant lasts depends on a lot of things, including the health of your eye and whether you have any other eye conditions, like a cataract or glaucoma. There are lots of people who have had their grafts for 10+ years without any problems.

But, nothing lasts forever, and a corneal transplant – just like everything in life – can wear out. If so, it can always be repeated.

87. Where do you get the donor corneal tissue from?

Your new cells come from a deceased person who was an organ donor.

88. Can you tell me about the donor that my corneal transplant is coming from?

There's some limited information that we can give you, like the age and sex of the person that your cells are coming from.

89. Can I pick my own donor tissue?

While it's not possible for you to pick your own tissue, rest assured that your doctor will be extremely careful to select only high-quality cells for your operation.

90. Can I still be an organ donor if have this surgery?

Yes! While your corneas would not be used again for another person, you can still be an organ donor.

91. Since the surgery, I've noticed that my eye feels scratchy sometimes. Is that normal?

Yes. Mild and occasional "dry eye" is very common as we get older, and after any eye surgery, including DMEK. Artificial tears should help some. However, if you feel like your eye is becoming more irritated, or the drops aren't working, you need to be examined by your eye doctor to make sure that there isn't something more serious going on (like a graft rejection).

92. Since the surgery, I've noticed that I can see a black dot on my eye. What is that?

During the surgery, we may create a tiny escape valve somewhere on your iris, which may be visible after your surgery as a little black dot. We do that to protect you from developing a high pressure after the operation. This little black dot is usually not visible to anyone (including the patient!). It does not usually go away on its own, but it does not hurt the eye.

93. My surgery was years ago, and everything has been fine, but lately my eye has been red and hurting. What should I do?

It could be dryness or allergy or any number of things, but you must go to your eye doctor and be examined – it's possible that your graft is rejecting, and if so, it needs to be treated, immediately.

94. How soon after the first eye can the second eye be operated on?

We always want the first eye to be your good eye before operating on the second one. Everyone heals differently but, in general, two weeks after the first surgery is the soonest we'd consider operating on your second eye.

95. After I have this surgery, does this mean I need to see a corneal specialist forever?

Probably not. Most people can go back to their regular eye doctor about a month after the surgery and only return to see a corneal specialist if they have a problem.

96. I've heard that Fuchs dystrophy can be treated in some patients by just scraping the back of the cornea, and not doing a transplant at all. Is that true, and if so, am I candidate for this procedure?

Rarely, this is true – just removing some of the diseased cells from the back of the cornea can be effective in some patients. Right now, this procedure remains experimental. If you want to know whether you might be a candidate for this type of operation, please ask your corneal specialist to discuss it with you.

97. Is there anything new coming up that would be better than DMEK? Should I wait?

   New stuff is coming out all the time. If you're not having any problems, there's probably no rush to have surgery. On the other hand, if you're having trouble, there's no reason for you to be stumbling around when DMEK has a good chance of making you a lot better off than you are now.

98. I'd like to donate to the research efforts of Dr. Melles. Where can I do that?

   To contribute, please visit https://www.mellesresearchfonds.nl/en/

99. Are there any other books on the subject of DMEK that I might find interesting or useful?

   We've written two other books about DMEK (mostly for other doctors). If you're really interested, or if you need something to read at night to put yourself quickly to sleep, you can find them on Amazon – just search "DMEK."

www.ingramcontent.com/pod-product-compliance
Lightning Source LLC
Chambersburg PA
CBHW040415220526
45473CB00004B/1249